# Prof P's Guide to Nursing School:
*Using tips, tricks, mindset & study habits.*

Mary Phillips MSN, RN

Prof P's Guide to Nursing School:
*Using tips, tricks, mindset & study habits.*

Mary Phillips MSN, RN

ISBN: 978-1-965016-07-7



Publishing Company: Platypus Publishing

# Contents

# Important Terms & Abbreviations

| | |
|---|---|
| NCLEX | National Council Licensure Examination |
| NCSBN | National Council of State Boards of Nursing |
| ANA | American Nurses Association |
| Next Gen | style of questions on the NCLEX that are updated and multifaceted |
| ADPIE | Assessment, Diagnosis, Plan, Intervention, Evaluation |
| mL | milliliter |
| G or g | gram |
| mg | milligram |
| mcg | microgram |
| L or l | liter |
| tsp | teaspoon |
| Tsp | tablespoon |
| oz | ounce |
| K or k | kilogram |
| lb | pound |
| 5mL | 1 teaspoon |
| 15mL | 1 Tablespoon |
| 1oz | 30mL |
| 1000mL | 1L |
| 1000mg | 1g |
| 1000mcg | 1mg |
| 1kg | 1000g |
| 1kg | 2.2lbs |

# Introduction

Tell me if this sounds familiar…

After several semesters of prerequisites, you complete your Nursing School application and begin the waiting game. Once the acceptance letter date rolls around, you refresh your inbox repeatedly, daily, repeatedly, hourly, repeatedly; look in your mailbox daily. The anticipation is so high you can hardly stand it. Then, on a random rainy day when you least expect it, "DING!" it's your email notification, and your letter is in your inbox! After opening the email, you read, YOU WERE ACCEPTED! The level of excitement and accomplishment makes you want to burst and shout, "I DID IT!"

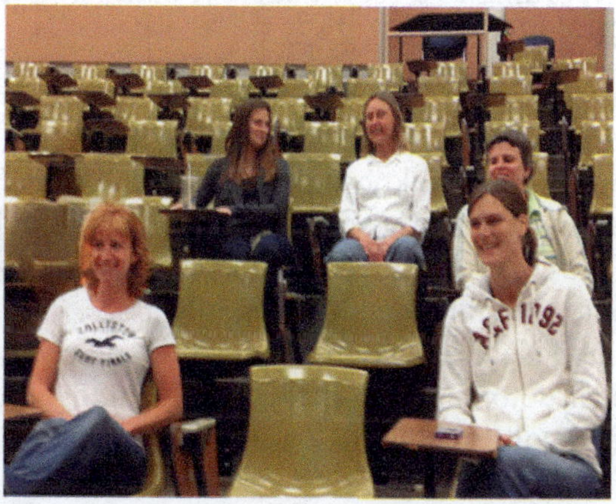

This level of energy is maintained for some time; the excitement lives on up to and including the sheer joy on the faces of students at Nursing Orientation (pictured). This occurs every year, faces go from these bright cheery expressions to pained, stressed, tired expressions that lack that initial excitement. Why does this happen?

After students accomplish their goal to enter Nursing School, why do they look like they lost their puppy to the streets, their spouse to a mob boss, or their best friend to being flattened by a bus?

After 11 years as a full time Nursing Professor at a community college and an additional 10 years of adjunct nursing education, I concluded that students lacked the belief that success does not have to be quite so difficult. Indeed, quite the opposite, the experience must match the career reputation of "being in the trenches," "burning the candle at both ends," "running ragged," to the point of being sick during each semester break. The badge of stress is carried almost with honor by those in nursing school. It is not a badge at all, it is a fast track to elevated cortisol levels that can lead to a slew of health issues. Not just nursing school but the entire field of nursing is wrought with stress and burnout, in fact, nearly two thirds of nurses experience it according to a recent survey, many of whom are only in their 20's (Sabei et al., 2022).

*Prof P's Guide to Nursing School Success* will help readers understand the importance of perspective and preparation. How would people know what to prepare for? The stories passed on are horror stories of trudging on and barely making it through. The set up begins even during prerequisite courses and bleeds into the start of core nursing classes. The expectation is that it is supposed to be awful, stressful, and painful. Not to mention the instructors, they must be old curmudgeons who are mean, strict, and cold! Right? Not exactly…

The students seemed to have this false belief that professors were eager for students to fail. On exam days, based on the level of stress observed, I incorporated many strategies, including writing positive affirmations that they would read before the exam or writing what your worry is on a paper and throwing it.

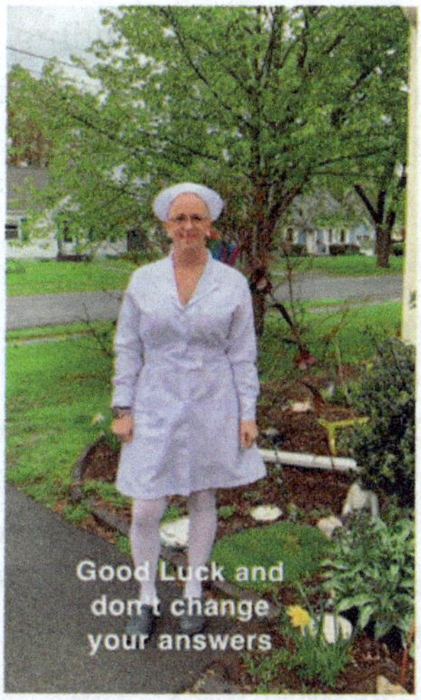


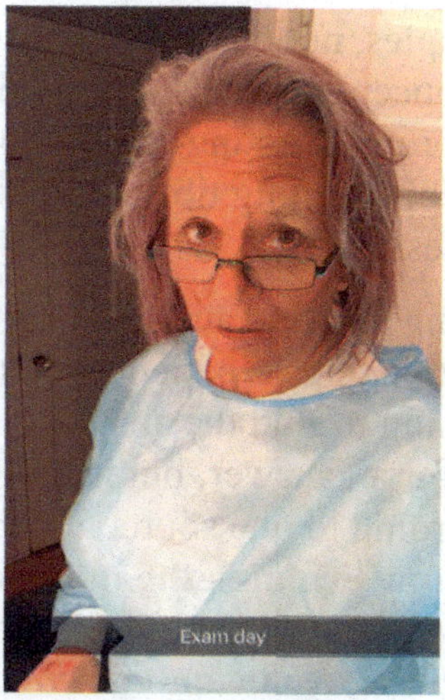


However, one strategy was born accidentally at the beginning of my full-time nursing education career and continued until retirement. Based on the buzz during the days leading to exam day, the stress was palpable. At one exam, I dressed in costume for Halloween, my favorite holiday, and I realized that students began asking me more about the costume than the exam for a few moments. Hence, I decided to make exam-day costumes a tradition.

Instructors stress over students who are not performing well. None of the instructors I knew were deliberately trying to make it impossible for students to achieve passing grades.

Perhaps the nature of prerequisite courses created this false belief. Many students used memorization to pass general education classes. However, memorization is not an effective mode of learning in nursing. Nursing classes require both specific facts and the procedural steps needed to demonstrate deep understanding of how to treat various diseases and injuries. Prof P's Guide to Success will help you apply effective learning principles, not only to pass a test, but for deep understanding of the concepts and skills needed to be an effective nurse. My goal is to provide testing-taking tips, organizational tips, and academic writing tips to avoid a sense of feeling lost and hopeless.

Finding answers and solutions with resources is what nursing does to navigate patients and the varied needs they have. Learning to find the answers is not something students like to hear for an answer, but it is the answer that best serves them. According to one source, "…here's the dangerous part: **when someone explains the material to you, you will *feel* like you know enough to think like a nurse, even though you really don't**. And you won't discover your error until the end of nursing school when you can't pass exit exams…or NCLEX." (Whitworth, 2024).

This guide will first explain how personality types and learning styles help you understand and shape the kind of student you are. This analysis will prevent feeling defeated if your learning style is different. Knowing your learning style and understanding what you need makes learning much easier. This book sets out to help you better prepare and understand the next steps.

Although some of these suggestions may seem like extra work, employing these suggestions will help reduce anxiety, which will itself help you think more clearly under pressure.

## Professor Phillips' Students' Comments

"She was personable, fun and humble. She tried to make us students relax around her, while other instructors made nursing school scary. She cared about all of us, shows how big her heart is." Aya Kotaich BSN, RN

“I lived in three different countries and in one I did not speak the language. I had to learn street smarts about who I could trust. From day one, she never gave me one red flag. What I saw is what I got, I treated her with respect and I can say she reciprocated that 100% and more.” Daniel Adjei ADN, RN

“She was honest, and compassionate, yet firm.” Julie Burke

“It was clear that she knew her information, she answered any question without judgment and she explained everything in real world experience so we could understand. Also she made a hard time being in school, fun.” Kayla Gilmore

“Her honest vulnerability was one reason I liked her and the depth of knowledge of her trade.” Jennifer Veccillio BSN, RN

“I feel incredibly fortunate to have had her as my Professor. Her unwavering support and encouragement meant everything to me and I am truly thankful. She was more than a professor to me; she was a mentor and a source of strength to continue following my future career path. The students and myself were very lucky to have had the privilege of learning from her.” Lenna T. (student)

## What to expect within this book

Each chapter has a sticky note icon that has a QR code that will link you to a personal message from me. Each message is tied directly to the topic of the chapter. Additionally, there are questions at the end of each chapter that will be thought provoking to aid you in considering key points or methods for you to explore to help you as a learner.

- **What are your biggest hurdles beginning nursing school?**
- **What are your expectations?**
- **Are your expectations realistic?**

# Chapter 1: Nursing School and Mindset

Think about how you approach hard things. Are you a bundle of nerves? A hot mess? The natural leader? The ostrich? All these responses are present in some form for each person. The predominant aspect steps forward during times of high stress.

"Psych Central identifies five types of personalities that, in part, define how people respond to stress" (Gepp et al., para 9, 2022).

- **Neuroticism**: emotional instability, self-consciousness
- **Extraversion**: seeks out excitement and social interactions
- **Openness**: creative, aesthetic, looks for new experiences
- **Agreeableness**: tends to be cooperative, trusting, gets along with others
- **Conscientiousness**: dutiful, competent, has a sense of purpose

Nursing school requires, among other elements, papers, projects, individual and group assignments, and exams. In my experience, when students enter an advanced educational program, without even realizing it, they become labeled “the leader” or “the peacemaker” or something that sounds a bit less competent. Do you have the “if I don’t do it, it won’t get done right” mindset? If so, you may be labeled a “control freak.” Are you prepared to go through school in that role? What if a crisis hits and you happen to be the one who needs help? How can you step away from being the leader? Do you believe no one else will get it done right and you will lose your A+ average?

Walking into any situation is always better when you are armed with knowledge that allows for informed decision making. Being a natural born leader is great if you are willing to be that leader. Some learners and a leader do the actual work so the lazy learner can focus on studying. A lazy group member might drag their feet so someone else does the work. These students apologize and make excuses but someone else does their work. Anyone who has done group work will have experienced this type of group member.

If you know your predominant role you can prevent yourself from taking on the entire project. Understanding your personality and how it propels you into roles helps you connect that to how you handle stress. “No matter what personality traits you identify with, it’s possible to adopt healthy and effective stress-coping strategies” (Gepp, Karin and Lovering, Cathy, para 15, 2022).

First, be an intentional self-advocate and be self-reflective. In a study group, are you the complainer? The problem solver? The sympathizer? The doer? Knowing and being honest with yourself is a good place to start.

Take this quiz to see your personality type:
https://www.truity.com/test/disc-personality-test

Take this quiz to see your learning style:
https://vark-learn.com/the-vark-questionnaire/

The old way of thinking about going to college includes questions like, what am I good at? what do I like doing? and what subjects are strong for me? According to *UWorld*, new research shows that, "For nursing students, embracing a growth mindset instead of a fixed mindset can significantly contribute to didactic, clinical, NCLEX®, and eventual career success." (UWorld LLC, 2023). UWorld discusses two mindsets, fixed and growth, para 6, 2023. Fixed mindsets are seemingly unmovable or unchangeable. This mindset is a limiting belief; believing that you have no control over your thinking is the first step to making things harder on yourself. Consider the superficial fallacy of this self-belief: if you could not grow or learn, would you be able to gain acceptance to Nursing School? The discrepancy between your self-concept and your achievement initiates the stress and struggle.

I have told students attending Nursing School Orientation that if they can learn to care for themselves and provide self-compassion in the same way they treat others, they would be miles ahead of their predecessors. Learning to set limits with others to advocate for what is needed is part of this bigger picture.

For example, Karen is a 23-year-old mother of two children, one two years old and one six months old, who goes into Nursing School. At orientation she learns that she will have clinical either two days a week for six hours each or one 12-hour clinical day; lab for three hours one day; and two two-hour classes per week. This course load comes on top of studying, scheduling Community Service as part of clinical, and working 24 hours a week, this all immediately sends her into stress-scheduling mode. Her partner does not support her decision to go to school. Although Karen stresses how much this will help them financially, her partner does not budge. In fact, her partner says that they will not take on any household duties, so she has to figure out how she is going to do the childcare and household tasks to prevent any problems while she is at school. She considers three options:

- Try to handle it all, not ask for help, and drown in stress
- Ask for a divorce (and drown in stress)
- Begin to evaluate how limits can be set to provide herself with support

While this seems like an extreme example, it is more common than you would imagine. This is Nursing; the people who enter this field tend to be caretaking individuals who are used to taking on a lot. I cannot enumerate the number of breakups, divorces, separations, and rough patches I have supported. Connecting with campus support, women's resources, and community support options often help.

Is the importance of mindset coming into focus? Does this mean if you have to do it all by yourself to succeed? It means success will be harder for you than for less-encumbered people. Sit your family down and make sure they know when you will be gone and how they can help. Have plans B and C because, well, life happens. Your coping mechanisms, problem-solving skills, and learning style contribute to finding a way to succeed that works for you. Knowing that learning by doing is as important for a kinetic learner as reading for understanding is for a visual learner will help you understand why some study methods work better for you.

If you have a support group, make sure they are aware of your schedule, but make sure you know how you best manage stress. Nursing is a stressful field. You will be distributing medications, treating injuries and illnesses, charting vital signs and other indications of improvement or decline, consoling families, and completing all the work tasks for multiple patients. Knowing how you manage stress will allow you to invoke those coping skills. Time management is key because building a ten-minute stress-relieving technique into your schedule will be a game changer for you. Running on stress is asking to become a patient!

Test anxiety (TA) is also part of the mindset and is more than believing in yourself. TA includes psychological and physical responses; the onus of managing TA falls on you. Seeking accommodations for extra time is one possible accommodation. It is important to get to the basics of how you operate effectively in a testing situation to uncover information about your learning type.

A systematic review of studies done about TA uncovered inconsistencies of interventions for decreasing TA (Kaur et al., 2023). While some students experienced a decrease in TA symptoms with aromatherapy and music, other results found guided imagery and other interventions helpful. One intervention can help some but annoy or interrupt other testers. One consideration is that aromatherapy can be harmful; it can trigger allergies, headaches, or nausea in some people. Music can distract some students, but soothe others. As a tester, you must identify what helps you and develop a plan to enlist the aid in a fashion that does not disturb or disrupt others.

*UWorld* provides a real-world NCLEX experience. The screen color, font, and timer are the same as in the actual NCLEX. Simple *UWorld* testing strategies (2023) include the following:

- Instead of saying "I suck at math," say "I am not as good at math as I would like." This tells your brain you believe you can do the work, but you need more practice.
- Do not block yourself into a failure mindset. For instance, "I am doing the work, but I am not getting it; maybe I shouldn't become a nurse." Instead of dead-end thinking, problem solve, make a plan, and think about problem-solving as a process. If you have to approach a problem from a different angle, walk away for a few moments to find some clarity about the solution.
- Stop using memorization as a learning method. It really is not the way to understand nursing concepts. Some can memorize concepts and turn them into practice, but it is not the norm. A growth mindset tackles learning through multiple means, persistence, collaboration, and creativity.
- For a particularly big assignment, exam, or project, instead of getting overwhelmed and experiencing brain freeze, approach preparation as a way to flex an undeveloped learning muscle.

After accomplishing a challenge, how many times do you reflect and think, "How did I ever do that? How did I find the time to fit that in?" When we set our minds to a task, we can usually do it even when we have serious doubts. So, task number one is to work on mindset. You do not have to put off school because you never focused on this before; taking mindset into consideration is already planting the seeds that you can do it and with less stress. Setbacks can happen, especially when deadlines loom.

Getting used to the style of exam questions and writing is a process. The key to overcoming setbacks is to give your mindset a reboot.

- **What is your mindset?**
- **What ways can a more positive mindset help you?**
- **Try to catch yourself describing things that are hard, too much, or can't do… and change it to I have room to improve this skill, this is a lot but I can do hard things.**

# Chapter 2: Self-Care

Now that there is perspective on how mindset plays a role in the success of a student, let's talk about self-care! Why is it the most important thing you can do for yourself? This is not only for the student portion of life but also the graduated novice nurse, experienced nurse, parent, partner, family, and friend portion of life. The point cannot be stressed enough,

The giving professions are especially susceptible to losing work-life balance. Giving constantly to everyone, as nurses tend to do, without taking time for self-care, often leads to burnout and bitterness, which affects one's entire life. In fact, the American Nurses Association (ANA) Code of Ethics mandates self-care.

"The fifth provision of the American Nurses Association's Code of Ethics states that the moral respect that nurses extend to all human beings should extend to themselves as well. These duties include the responsibility to:

- Promote health and safety

- Preserve wholeness of character and integrity
- Maintain competence
- Continue personal and professional growth

"The nurse owes the same duties to self as to others, including the responsibility to promote health and safety, preserve wholeness of character and integrity, maintain competence, and continue personal and professional growth." (Purdue, para 7, 2024)

Imagine the following scenario. Before you leave for work, you and your spouse fight about the bills; your two-year old is sick and you have to find a place for her because her regular daycare won't take her; and you get stopped for speeding. Your shift begins. You have six patients; two require two-person assists, and one is on hourly vital-signs monitoring. You have to manage medication passes, treatments, getting the patients to and from tests, family concerns, doctors' orders and requests, and the dynamics of the unit you work on. While you make your rounds to each patient, you discover one of them on the floor, and after assessment, the patient may have a fracture. When you speak with the family, the daughter begins crying and blaming you. You remain on the phone with her although you have scheduled medications to administer and treatments to perform. Next, the nursing supervisor asks you to stay four more hours due to a sick call for the next shift.

Do you need a deep breath? I do!

This is a typical example of a day in the life of a nurse based on real-life examples shared by friends, students, and coworkers. If this level of stress goes unaddressed, where will your compassion and empathy come from?

Learning to be compassionate with ourselves is important for everyone, but it is especially important for those of us who give by caring for those around us.

Building and prioritizing a practice of self-care requires knowing how to fill your cup after a day of depletion. You need to factor self-care into your schedule. Think about the activities that allow you to relax, move your body, and laugh. While you probably can't fit in multiple self-care activities every day, consider prioritizing one or two things that will really help in that moment. Think about combining simple activities, such as walking while listening to a good book or enjoying a sweet bedtime routine with your children. Sometimes, it's all about attitude; finishing a simple task can result in a sense of relaxation.

If you can set aside a certain amount of time for dedicated self-care, fill a jar with notes with different options for meeting your needs instead of scheduling something predictable. Write 10 suggestions for each category (physical, mental, spiritual, etc.) and mix all the papers in the jar. Pull a paper every day during your allotted self-care time. Once you complete an activity, place the note in a completed jar. Keep adding to your self-care jar, be kind, and feel free to pull a different note if one does not appeal to you. Notice that doing nothing can be self-care if you call it "meditation."

The World Health Organization (WHO) also supports self-care for healthcare workers. "In the case of nurses, self-care means taking action to reduce stress and take care of one's own physical, mental, emotional, and spiritual needs. Rather than viewing self-care as an occasional indulgence, nurses should consider self-care as a pillar of preventive care" (Bradley University, para 4, 2024).

Bradley University takes self-care to the level of including things like travel and creative expression (2024). Does painting calm you? Dancing? Running? Crocheting? The self-care plan is similar to a plan of care for a patient. You can partake in an activity and then note how you feel when you finish it. If you notice a decrease in stress or increase in focus, incorporate more of that during those designated self-care time slots.

Self-care applies just as importantly to nursing school. You may not have a floor full of patients, but you have a calendar full of assignments, clinicals, community work, studying, and the demands of your family. Self-care can be as simple as getting proper sleep, diet, and exercise; establishing a peer or friend group; meditating; going outdoors; and decompressing at the end of the day (Concordia University Texas, 2024).

"Here are a few ways you can create personal time in your nursing school schedule and decompress:

- Start by setting aside an hour a day for a leisure activity. Adjust the length based on how much time you need for studying each day.
- Add breaks to your schedule, and don't skip them. Prioritize this time for your mental wellness.
- Make a list of your top priorities, and spend time on them. Cut out activities that don't add value to your life.
- Write in a journal before bed.
- Listen to music or a favorite podcast as you get ready for bed.
- Read a chapter in a non-nursing book before falling asleep." (Concordia University Texas, 2024)

Do you see the pattern? Simple and small changes can impact your ability to recuperate and rejuvenate!

- **What are your take-aways for self-care?**
- **List three changes or additions you will make to increase your self-care.**

# Chapter 3: Professionalism

While this may seem like a no-brainer, I assure you that it is not. There is a range in which students have experience in communicating, though in most cases, who are they communicating most with? Family, friends, co-workers and maybe bosses. The number of text messages and emails received as a professor that did not address anyone or have a closing salutation was staggering. It generally took a conversation and sometimes being written up before a student would take the professor seriously.

The following list provides some main points.

- Do not use text slang and abbreviations such as R (are), U (you), TY (thank you), B4 (before), etc. This short-hand notation should be reserved for friends and family.

- Open and close a text or an email with a greeting and close the communication with your name. This is basic professionalism for all forms of written business communication.
- Identify yourself in text messages. Most instructors who allow students to text do not save students' contact information in their phones.

The following list provides guidelines for solving more difficult or sensitive problems.

- No matter with whom or what, remain relentlessly polite and calm. Nothing will be gained with any other approach. Define the problem and identify your part rather than blaming anyone else. Focus on finding a realistic solution, not necessarily the one you want.
- Follow the "chain of command" and begin with the person the challenge is with. For example, if you struggle with your clinical instructor, do not skip to the president of the college to help resolve it. Only escalate up the chain if there is no other recourse. Attempting to usurp the system will reflect negatively on you. Following the chain of command and leveraging system resources will earn you respect for dealing with the issue at hand with the person most able to help you find a solution. You will demonstrate your professionalism and your logical approach to problem solving and conflict resolution.
- Do not expect that every issue you have will result in your preferred solution. Approach each issue with detached curiosity rather than accusing or blaming the other person. For example, if the issue is over a disappointing grade on an

assignment, consider asking the instructor to explain the deficiency and how you can improve.

Evaluations are a chance for professors to provide constructive feedback, but they have to observe regulations and time constraints. Politely ask for an appointment and more detailed information about what went wrong and how *you* can do better. Was your logic off course? Did you base an answer on an incorrect interpretation of a scenario? If you focus your appointment on getting help rather than accusing the professor of negligence or incompetence, you may find your instructor noticing a lack of clarity in a question resulting in a change in your favor. One of the best results, regardless of the academic impact on this particular assignment, is that you'll walk away with your instructor's high opinion of your ability to negotiate conflict situations. Ultimately, recognize that you are responsible for your own successes and mistakes.

- Adhere to due dates and do not expect that every request for extensions will be granted. Instructors are very likely to realize when such a request is due to a lack of planning versus an emergent or unexpected reason.

Entering the healthcare field is not unlike other jobs for professional communications with clients and co-workers. Though the level of interprofessional communication requires the utmost in professionalism because the documentation and communication between professionals is subject to litigation if there is a poor patient outcome. Therefore, nurses should not respond to patients or colleagues with "dude, that blood pressure is high!" or "wow dawg, that wound looks gnarly!" Speaking and writing professionally means communication is taken seriously. Those written words turn into financial reimbursement from insurance companies and can prevent nurses from litigation. “There is a huge liability issue that can occur when care documentation is inaccurate or if the documentation reflects unclear information.” (Wong, C., 2023). Documentation that is clear and accurate paints a clear picture for other providers and the court if a case does go to litigation.

Note the following examples of documentation.

> **Incorrect and unclear:** Client reported pain in the left arm, red spot noted by the elbow, warm to touch, doctor notified.

> **Correct and clear:** Client reported pain 2/10 on the pain scale and tingling in their left arm on the anterior portion. Along the seam of the temporary cast, 3 cm proximal to the elbow, is a blanchable red area 2 cm by 3.5 cm. The area is slightly warm to touch. The patient reports relief when the temporary cast is adjusted and lined with lambswool at that location. Reported to MD, no new orders at this time, will continue to monitor twice a shift, nursing order entered into treatment book.

Documenting clearly is crucial in capturing the good patient care that is delivered in part for reimbursement as mentioned but also, as important is the possibility of litigation in nursing, the documentation needs to be legible, accurate, and clear. This leaves zero question about what was done on what and where paints a clear trail of care. It is a good idea to have a coworker or supervisor on the scene read a note based on a challenging or difficult patient to verify that the language is objective. Collaboration in healthcare is important, and a second set of eyes that knows the situation can help ensure that the note is clear, complete, and accurate.

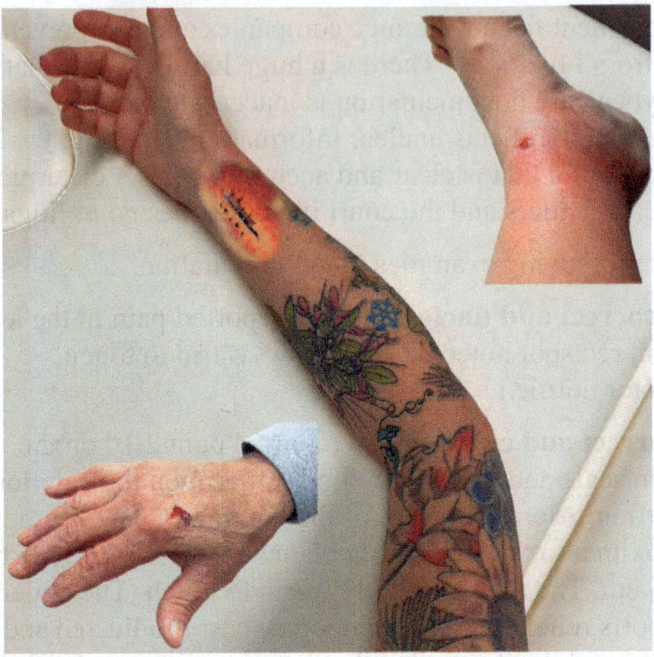

- **Document with as much detail and descriptors for the assessment on the hand, arm or leg. Consider location and the issue.**
- **What will the documentation need to include to be clear?**

# Chapter 4: Study Habits for Success

## Learning, Study Habits, and Time Management

I mentioned previously that memorization is not the preferred way to learn nursing information. Flash cards can help with terminology in various classes, but they won't help you think through a solution to a problem. An age-old joke about nurses says, "Nurses make lists and then a list from the list and usually color coded." To a certain extent, this is true, especially the color coding. I encourage the following practices:

- Make a list of the work you have due each day. Use color codes to help organize and prioritize. For example: write exams in pink, papers in green, and practice quizzes or lab assignments in yellow or blue, respectively. Make this list in order of required dates. When studying for exams, pick up a notebook and pen or pencil and write, write, write. Itemize each key topic and subtopics. What your professor is highlighting for this test. Use the unit outline to make notes from your textbook and lecture notes. You may be able to trade notes with a fellow student as you study together.

- From the notes, make study cards with short anecdotes or drawings to help the visual recall the information.
- During classes record the lectures (if it is allowed) and listen again while driving. This is an excellent way to learn and let it sink in, especially for auditory learners.

The more you write out the information, the more likely it will stick in your brain. Haury, a blogger, writes in the study conducted by a duo, "this repetitive, creative handwriting also creates stronger reading comprehension and maturity of language recognition" (Haury, C., para 7, 2022). Writing is a form of visual and kinesthetic learning because of the physical formation of the letters and words. This concept further strengthens the idea that the written word is linked to building a foundation of recall. Haury further notes that writing by hand, due to its visual nature, highlights the information and paints a picture for your brain to recall (Haury, C. 2022).

While typing or taking notes on your smartphone or tablet seems like it might accomplish the same thing, it does not. "Digital tools have uniform scrolling up and down and standardized arrangement of text and picture size, like on a webpage. If you remember a physical textbook printed on paper, you can close your eyes and visualize the photo one-third of the way down on the left-side page and the notes you added in the bottom margin" (Haury, para 10, 2022). "Your writing, your shorthand, and your notes that look incomprehensible to others are a special part of your processing that help you learn in your way" (Haury, para 15, 2022).

Learning or relearning cursive handwriting might feel difficult and inefficient, but it will become easier over time, especially when you start seeing results. Grabbing your pencil or pen to take notes versus using your smartphone will take practice, but eventually you will develop a routine. DePaul notes that a habit is a behavior done with little or no thought (not especially helpful for learning), while a routine involves a series of behaviors frequently and intentionally repeated. A behavior has to be a regularly performed routine before it can become a habit (DePaul et al., 2021, para 6).

## Study Groups

Study groups are a recommended technique for learning new information. The scheduled routine and interchange of questions and explanations help embed knowledge. However, knowing how you learn best is important. If you are easily distracted or confused by listening to others, a small group may be best for you. Speedyprep (2022) notes that study groups are successful learning tools due to the following:

- **Procrastination Solution**. Knowing you have a regularly scheduled study session means you need to be prepared to make your participation worth your time. Showing up unprepared will likely annoy or upset others who are ready to learn.

- **Learn Faster**. Each person in the group contributes different perspectives and levels of understanding. While one member may be confused by a topic, another might understand it easily. The sharing of this knowledge benefits everyone. The confused student gets examples from a fellow student's perspective, while the student who knows it solidifies their sense of the topic by putting it into words to help their friends understand.

- **New Perspective**. Hearing other students' examples of how they see the topic or how they understand the material triggers your critical thinking skills as you compare your understanding of the topic to what others share. The more perspectives that help clarify a topic, the wider the understanding for the group.
- **Learn new study skills**. Listening to others' perspectives in a group can add to your study skills base and broaden your perspective on how you think about the topic.
- **Variety is the spice…** When you have only your perspective, thoughts, and habits, you can be more distractible and less focused. Moving to a different scene boosts your brain, study abilities, and content comprehension.
- **Real-life practice**. Studying with other classmates in a group setting will stretch your people skills. We do not all think alike or view things the same, so by sharing information, your people skills naturally grow. If for no other reason, navigating studying under some stress forces us to develop healthy coping skills for when we are on the floor working with others.

"There are no shortcuts, no secret formula," Mandibaya said. "But being in a study group gave all of us an edge" (Chamberlain University, para 1, 2023). Establishing boundaries for study groups is a key concept. If the group is too large, confusion can occur. Additionally, using a group session to criticize the instructor or program is not helpful. Your family and friends can be the sounding board for such things.

Dedicating the study group for studying benefits all participants. Designating a focus topic with everyone arriving with their questions about the topic helps to keep the information flowing. Specifying an entire unit for exam prep is helpful. Everyone can bring their points of confusion, and the group can discuss and help each other. It is rare that every person is confused about the same topic; magic happens when each member shares their understanding of a given topic. When a student or tutor re-words concepts in their own understanding, lightbulbs go off for others who may be confused.

Breaking up with my study group, is that a thing? Yes, it is! If the group is not productive, or is too chatty making it hard for learning, it is crucial for you to state this to the group and politely excuse yourself from the sessions. While this may be hard or awkward, you will be advocating for patients and or yourself with staffing or workload so getting used to communicating your needs is super important. If it is too hard to be honest, you can always bow out with a 'time conflict' excuse. The long and short of it is learning to use your voice. In nursing we must advocate for patient care, family support, discharge planning and teamwork. All of these things may require a voice capable of setting boundaries. Hence the reason to begin during school to increase your familiarity and capability of doing so.

## Practice Questions

First of all, DO NOT USE QUIZLET! It does not teach or help you do anything but memorize. Memorization in nursing is only useful if you are studying lists of things such as medications in a pharmacologic class or the nerves in the spinal cord. To develop a true understanding of the material requires a clear understanding of the topic so that the concept can be transferred to multiple scenarios.

For example: Blanchability of skin. If the patient is bed-bound, you may note redness on the coccyx, heels, or spine from extended contact with the bed. Without a clear understanding of what blanching or a lack of it means, the nurse will miss the signs of skin breakdown. Due to the lack of understanding and knowledge of the remedy, the nurse will allow the patient to remain in the same position, further damaging the area. Memorizing the definition of blanchability allows you to remember that blanching it is good, but not what to do if blanching does not occur or the appropriate interventions.

If your school is a quality nursing program, accredited and such, they will be creating their own questions further making Quizlet useless. A good program has instructors who are trained to create their own NCLEX style questions and new Next Generation questions. The study tips and test-taking tips for these will come later.

Use your resources to study the topics at hand with practice questions that have rationales for the incorrect and correct answers. While rationales can explain the answers that are wrong, it is important to know why an answer is right. If you happen to guess correctly or are recalling it from your notes, you might not be able to synthesize the reason for this intervention, medication, or procedure for other types of needs. These practice questions are often found at the end of your chapters and in supporting materials.

Practice the question style you are weakest at. If Select All That Apply (SATA) questions are your nemesis, do those until you get them. These questions require you to know the material as a concept and remember the information and its use in multiple situations. The Next Generation (Next Gen) questions require multiple levels of thought and pulling it all together to get to the correct answer(s). Chapter 5 provides specific tips on these questions.

Relistening to the lecture is the most effective method for helping some students go from failing tests to passing with confidence. The dynamic is similar to watching a movie for the second or third time, when you notice details and continuity errors you missed the first time. Dr. Khanna explains, "Watching the same shows over and over again brings some sort of safety and comfort on a permanent level. It instills [sic] a sense of security, warmth, or wellbeing." She adds, "People also tend to watch the same shows and movies because that negates the feeling of disappointment and dissatisfaction. When you're tired, these familiar shows help you re-energize and restore the feeling of self-control. Especially when you're anxious" (Shah, para 9, 2022).

According to Richmond (2024) relistening to lectures is helpful for a number of reasons, which include

- The flexibility of relistening to cover the topic at your personal pace
- Enhancing the retention of information and the ability to fully understand a challenging topic
- Revisiting concepts and content for future exams or assignments

Nursing vocabulary and rationales are not like those in other general courses. Besides the ability to relisten to challenging sections of a given topic, noting the time of a hard topic in the recording creates a reference to the digital occurrence of that topic and makes it easier to find the section without having to relisten to the entire thing. Shah notes that recording the lecture reduces stress by knowing that you can actively listen to the material again (2022). Active listening focuses your full attention on the information and not on need to write frantically to get it all. Of course, make sure recording is allowed at your institution and seek permission for the individual instructor.

Recording should not take the place of attending class. Your physical presence in the classroom allows you to hear the information first hand and to participate in active learning exercises that occur during the class to reinforce the information. Just listening to the lecture is never intended as a way to replace live learning. Shah notes that the benefit of actively participating reinforces material that listening alone excludes (2022). Active participation is especially important for students who learn best by doing, this is probably true for most people even if they do not like it.

- **What way do you study best?**
- **What resources do you have to help you?**
- **Do you need or have a back-up plan for class and clinical?**
- **What are your top take-aways from this chapter?**

# Chapter 5: Nursing Writing Assignments

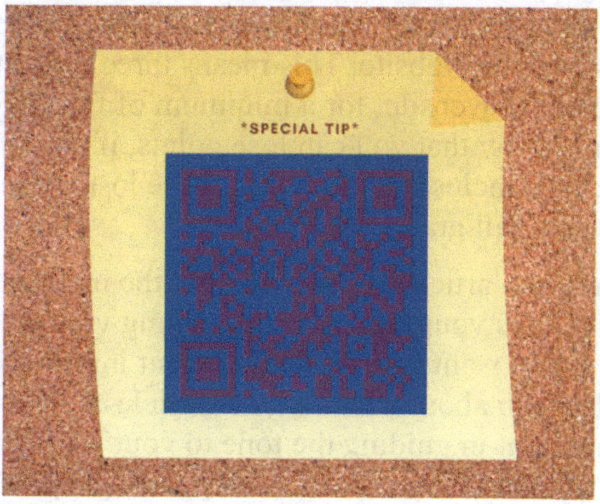


Writing a student paper in nursing is very different from writing a paper for English Literature or creative writing. A nursing paper must be evidence-based, professional, and with zero plagiarism. It is not to say that any other course allows plagiarism, however, given the level of integrity required in nursing, it is crucial to have sound information that is either clearly stated or cited properly. To write a nursing paper, select a topic appropriate to the assignment and then find supporting articles, ideally in a nursing database like CINHAL. The writing style needs to be formal, not "text-ese." Spell out contractions such as don't (do not) and they're (they are). Develop an outline to help structure the content and use the grading rubric to guide the focus and level of detail required for the paper.

The grading rubric is a blueprint of what to include in the paper. If the instructor does not have a rubric, ask them what guidelines will be used for grading. Additionally, the rubric should be in the course syllabus as well. Why you ask? The rubric may specify the inclusion of three sources published within the last seven years and one website. This means three separate articles on the topic plus a website, for a minimum of four references. This is a minor way that you can lose points, if you missed the required website inclusion, those points are lost, therefore, affecting the overall grade.

When you read an article, decide whether the information supports or refutes your thinking. Debunking viewpoints can be a reference if you want to provide divergent information. Making a decision about whether your articles will support or refute is important in guiding the tone to your writing. Debunking a point is fine as well as supporting a point, as long as you have the proof, aka the supporting data from the article to strengthen the paper's stance.

If you can print a copy of the article, make sure to include the bibliographic information for the citations and reference list. With a copy, you can highlight passages that you will paraphrase or quote directly. If you cannot print the article, start a page in your notebook, record the bibliographic source, and note key passages for paraphrasing or quotation. As you take notes, consider drafting your own paragraphs to include in your paper as ideas occur to you. It will speed up the writing process.

## Writing the Introduction

The introduction to a paper tells the reader about the paper and how the information will unfold. This helps the reader because it sets them up with how the paper will flow. For a paper about fruits and their health benefits, the introduction sets up the paper by introducing the reasons people find fruits beneficial and then includes the fruits in the order they appear in the paper.

For example:

> *Fruits in your diet are more than just yummy treats. The benefits may be surprising to you. Beyond the sweet taste of fruits, which can make vitamins and antioxidants a delicious addition to your diet, there are also a multitude of other benefits to your skin, body, and potential babies a woman may carry. Did you know that fruits may decrease cholesterol too? Fruits are seriously more than just a tasty treat. Leslie Barrie in Everyday Health 1996-2024 notes that the benefits include the addition of fiber, providing essential vitamins and antioxidants along. The following will cover the benefits and reasons for what fruits are the most beneficial, how to include them in your diet, and why it helps your body. (Phillips, M., 2024)*

This simplistic example allows the reader to know that the paper will cover the types of fruits that can be added to your diet, how to incorporate them, and their benefits. With an introduction like this, the reader will not be surprised at the unfolding of the paper. If the reader sees the introduction open with the benefits, the first paragraph after the introduction is not going to be where to find them. In the following example, more related to nursing school, skin breakdown is the assigned topic.

> *Nurses have many things that require attention throughout a work day. Patients' intake, output, vital signs, labs, tests, physical ability, medications,*

*treatments, and shift assessments. Among these tasks nurses will also be prioritizing the patients they are assigned to. Completing a head-to-toe shift assessment is among the first things to complete. During this process one the most preventable issues that can result from prolonged immobility or even decreased mobility is skin breakdown. Skin breakdown, aka pressure injuries result from many things but one common way is a lack of circulation to a given area that has pressure applied to it (Ahmad et al., 2023). Leading nursing responsibilities include skin assessment, pressure injury prevention, and treatment (Phillips, 2024).*

*This basic introduction leads the reader to conclude that assessment is first and foremost, because without identifying if a condition is an issue prevents the nurse from making evidence-based decisions for next steps. Assessment is followed by pressure injury prevention, and treatment. These actions, along with the evidence to support each aspect, provides the writer with a framework for the paper. The first section after the introduction will be the assessment of and identification of any problem areas, mobility issues, and the level of help the patient requires. Using the articles to support the writer in the assessment steps, strengthens the paper, identifies the types of prevention required, and allows the interventions needed to be developed informing the reader with solid data to practice with.*

Professional nursing papers are usually written in APA format. This tends to stress nursing students because they are not familiar with structured writing practices. There are helpful resources to aid the writer in maintaining the correct format.

Programs can be purchased, but the extra expense may be difficult for most college students. Capitalizing on free resources makes the most sense. I recommend the Purdue Owl website for instructors and students. This gives clear examples of reference pages and citations, paper set up, and APA rules in example format (Purdue Owl, 2024).

## Writing the Conclusion

The conclusion, like the introduction, clarifies and summarizes the main points of the paper. Include points made from your sources to strengthen your argument. For example:

> *Fruits in your diet are more than just yummy treats. Beyond being a sweet snack, they contain vitamins and antioxidants, making fruit not only beneficial to your body but to your skin, and pregnancies. Something the research lacked was more specific data regarding fruits and vegetables that may be helpful to all groups of people or if there is a cultural background that responds better or not as well as others. Being able to provide well rounded data is more directive for those who are looking to reap the benefits.*

This is a simplistic example of a conclusion; this is not the place to make new points or draw conclusions that are not supported in your paper. Inclusion of future needs for research is an excellent way to help wrap up your research, even if it means more the research has yet to be done.

## References and Citations

In writing your reference page, check the types of your resources, including books, web pages, journal articles, and educational sources. Find examples of references that use the prescribed format required by your instructor. The correct format is to list references in alphabetical order according to the author's last names. if you list a resource, you must use the source within the paper. Whether you include a direct quote, a paraphrase, or a summation to strengthen your point or hypothesis, be sure to cite your reference and list the references for your citations.

When you choose your rcferences, decide if you want to prove or disprove the stance taken within the paper, or if you want to show both sides of an argument and allow readers to decide for themselves. As you research your topic, the best approach will reveal itself to you. Writers learn different approaches to support or refute arguments that were initially known or thought. This kind of discovery is a powerful learning experience and can contribute to a strong conclusion.

It is not realistic to ask your instructor to pre-read your papers because that service would have to be offered to everyone; however, you should be able to meet with your professor to ask pointed questions and clarify what is expected. You can also use resources like your school library and peer tutor center. If your instructor does not require peer editing, you can still ask a classmate or another program participant who has done the assignment to read your paper and provide feedback. Provide your editor with the grading rubric and the assignment basics so they can provide more informed feedback. Using the grading rubric as a map to success is the best way to be sure you are on the right track.

- **What are your writing strengths?**
- **What do you need to improve?**

- **Where will you look for writing help?**

# Chapter 6: Test-Taking Tips

One of the unique things about nursing exams that make them different from other course exams is partly because all the answers to some questions are correct, but one or more answers can be considered *more* correct. The idea behind this 'diabolical' approach is to elicit the test-takers' critical thinking skills and reveal their thought processes. "Entry-level nurses are required to make increasingly complex decisions while delivering client care. These increasingly complex decisions often require the use of clinical judgment to support client safety. It is essential to note that clinical judgment applied in this dynamic supports the entry-level nurse to make effective decisions inside the nursing scope of practice, which provides a foundation for client safety. NCSBN has conducted several years of research and study to understand and isolate the individual factors that contribute to the process of nursing clinical judgment. These isolated factors are represented in the NCLEX-RN Test Plan and subsequently delivered as examination items" (NCSBN, section II para 3, 2023).

The NCSBN uses Computerized Adaptive Testing for the state board exam, and up to 19% of the questions can be centered on Pharmacology (NCSBN, 2023). This style of testing makes each exam specific to the tester because it adapts to what the tester knows and does not know to help determine their level of safety and ultimately their ability to become a nurse.

The nursing-school test plan has evolved over time and has become more complex in its ability to assess knowledge and judgment. The test had to evolve and grow in difficulty as the patient population has gotten sicker and more complex. The kinds of questions with answers that differ only slightly have frustrated students for as long as I taught nursing and far back as my training.

Practicing this style of testing allows students to develop their critical thinking abilities. Throughout a program, the exam will evolve from a greater ratio of knowledge-based questions to more advanced and complex questions that require information processing and a higher order of thinking. While research shows that changing answers is not proven to result in lower grades, the research is specific to changing answers because they mis-read the question or they found the correct answer later in the exam (Bauer et al, 2007). The following information explains why it is important to not change answers.

In a good nursing program, instructors create unique exam questions and do not use questions from a book or question bank. Good programs also use a framework to develop their exams. The main framework used in nursing is Bloom's Taxonomy (Ross, 2019). Beginning at the base (remember), these questions are knowledge-based questions and require memorized information. Lab values, medications and their uses, and signs and symptoms of a medical diagnosis are all examples of knowledge-based questions.

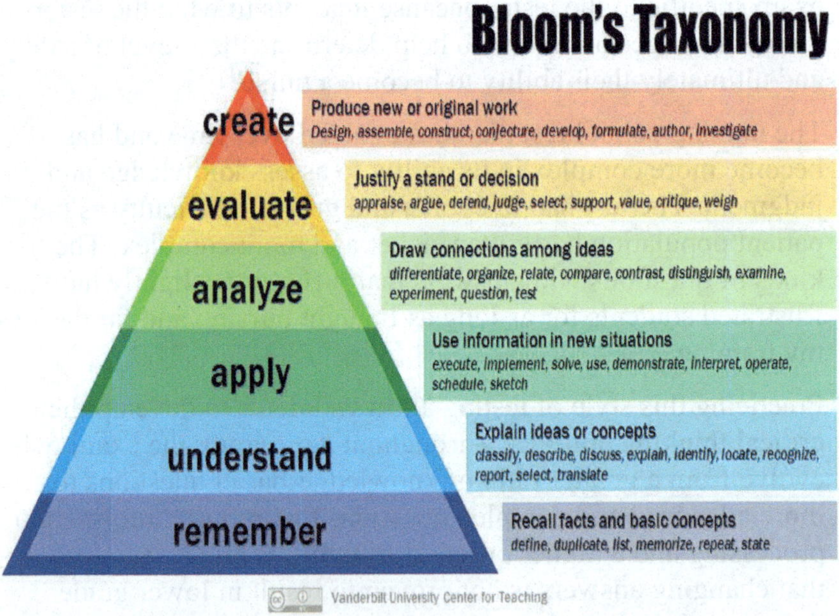


As the pyramid narrows towards the top, the types of questions and required knowledge grow in difficulty and become higher order types of situations or scenarios within a question, although one level of the pyramid can be embedded within another. For instance, a question about interventions for a client on a diuretic may contain portions that require recalling that a diuretic can lower blood pressure and require the reader to realize that lung sounds can reveal as much about the efficacy of the medication as blood pressure. This complex question elevates the questions from knowledge application because the reader must remember the drug class, the associated nursing actions, and determine the most correct answer based on the scenario posed in the question.

These complex questions incorporate the nursing process, or Assessment, Diagnosis, Plan, Implement, Evaluation (ADPIE) (Nugent & Vitale, 2021-22). The nursing process informs nursing decisions on almost every level. Whether you are doing an assessment or taking an exam, considering your full assessment allows you to develop a thought process about the diagnosis and develop a treatment plan. Implementing interventions to address patient needs and evaluate the plan's effectiveness is similar to the process required for taking an exam. You must read the question (Assessment), determine what it is asking (Diagnosis), read the answers (Plan), choose an answer (Implement), and then see how you did on the exam (Evaluation). While this is broken down for simplicity's sake, it will help you view all your decisions about patient care through the lens of the nursing process, even on exams.

## Nursing Process Approach to Exam Questions

- Assessment relates to data collection and forming an answer based on the data.
- Diagnosis or (as Nugent/Vitale write, 2021-2022) Analysis. This is one of the most challenging because so much has to be done to determine if a nursing diagnosis is to be made.

This may require data clustering to decide next steps.

- Planning as it relates to answering questions requires identifying the goal, listing or considering expected outcomes, prioritization and determining other members of the healthcare team for collaboration to plan the best course of action.
- Implementation requires data analysis with respect to the planning process to direct the interventions toward patient goals. Data, as it relates to legal parameters such as who is doing the assessing or interventions in the question, is a factor. Independent interventions are those the nurse can do alone without any input from a provider. If it is any other type of intervention, dependent interventions requiring a provider's order and interdependent aka collaborative interventions that are developed in conjunction with another professional (Nugent, P & Vitale, B. 2023-2024).
- Evaluation is the result of the complete nursing process through which the nurse determines if the interventions developed are accomplishing the steps toward goal attainment.

These methods or suggestions are not meant to be a failsafe guarantee that you will absolutely pass exams. These suggestions are meant to help you understand each question type and how to analyze them. Preparation is not solely about nursing knowledge but about yourself and how you learn, process information and ultimately practice in the profession.

**Dos:**

- Get a good night's sleep.
- Hydrate
- Eat a snack or a light meal before exams.
- Be on time! Rushing into a high-stakes test never ends well; you do not need additional stress on exam day.
- Exercise before the exam, even if only power walking for 10 minutes.
- When doing practice tests, limit yourself to one minute for each question.
- Manage your anxiety with one or more of the following techniques
    - Breathing techniques
    - Brushing to lower cortisol (Berg, E. MD, 2014)
    - Positive self-talk

- Read the entire question carefully while using your hand or a paper to cover the answers.
    - Take a deep breath
    - Reread the question
    - Answer the question in your mind before looking at the answers.
- Decide what the question is asking; it may help to mentally rephrase the question.
- Consider the time frame for the situation in the question; for example, postoperative day one, postpartum day one, or one hour after surgery.
- If prioritization is needed, identify the associated framework, such as Nursing Process, Maslow's Hierarchy of Needs, Kubler-Ross's Theory of Death and Dying, and apply the related principles to help answer the question (Nugent& Vitale 2012, 2023-2024).
- Answer the question in your head before looking at the answers.
- Read all the answers.
- Choose the best answer or answers.
- Make sure the answer makes sense.

**Don'ts:**

- Do not change your answer unless you read the question wrong. In all the years of teaching and exam reviews, the anecdotal data shows that innumerable students could have scored between 2 and 16 points more on their exam but because they changed their first correct answer to an incorrect one, they lost those points. Were there times that someone changed their answer and it was to the correct answer, of course, but predominantly this was not the case.

- Do not rely on word recognition. If you practiced questions about the heart that involved apical pulse, and the exam asks a question about a diuretic as a blood pressure medication, an apical pulse option in the answers is incorrect. Although it is customary to take an apical pulse for blood pressure medications, this particular question asks about how to determine if the medication is helping with congestive heart failure (CHF), the correct answer is to assess lung sounds to determine if the diuretic is helping to manage fluid overload.
- Do not stay too long on any question. If you are stuck, flag the question or write the question number on your scratch paper and go back to it later. If you are well prepared for the exam, most of the questions will be easy for you and you will have time to go back to the questions that you were struggling with. Also, the wording of other exam questions may shed light on the topic.
- Do not try to add or remove information in a question. Read the whole question and determine what it is asking. Do not think, "We did this in clinical," or "my mom had that." Trying to fit the question scenario into another one can be misleading. Focus on what the question is asking.
- Dismissive or falsely optimistic answer options are generally not correct because they can invalidate the patient's feelings. For example, if a patient is crying and the nurse states, "do not cry, all will be ok."

## Question Types

The previous guidelines on the dos and don’ts are general test-taking suggestions, but the question style often requires a deeper look. The best advice is to practice the style that is hardest for you.

The following information defines and describes the types of questions that can appear on an exam and provides strategies for understanding and answering each type.

### Multiple Choice

Multiple choice questions have two parts, a stem or the question and the answer options. As was previously mentioned, several answers *could* be correct; however, only one is actually correct. The options that are less correct or incorrect are called distractors, which are meant to tempt testers to require critical thinking to determine the correct answer. The best way to answer a traditional multiple-choice question is to use all the do’s and don'ts from above and to consider the following. Point words that make a question positive or negative should be in either underlined, italics, bold, or capital letters. Similar options that could both be correct require the If-Then method. Think, “if I do this intervention, then the outcome will be *xyz*. Extremely similar are generally not correct. If you can eliminate two choices from the list of answers, you narrow the choice of correct answer to a 50% chance that one of the two choices is correct (Nugent & Vitale, 2012). This information applies to regular multiple-choice questions that have only one answer, not another style that has multiple answers.

Some other strategies for plain multiple-choice questions include

- Decide if the question is about the nurse or the patient.
- Is the question asking for a particular aspect of ADPIE?
- If there are answers that are opposites, one of them is likely the answer.
- If more than one answer is very similar to another, both are usually incorrect.
- Answer choices that include *always, never*, or *none* are generally not correct.
- Assess whether the question is looking for a positive or negative response i.e., safest, first, best, or priority, compared to avoid, violate(s), never.
- Determine if the choices deny the client's feelings or needs.
- Do not diverge into another topic, focus on the question. Incorporate multiple techniques to answer the question.

**Multiple Response – Select all that apply**

Select all that apply (SATA) is a variation of multiple-choice questions that has one or *more* correct answers, up to all the choices being correct. The National Council of State Board of Nursing (NCSBN) has changed its stance on this in recent years (NCSBN, 2024). According to UWorld, SATA questions can have a single answer, but the NCSBN stance was that at least two correct answers were required (UWorld, 2021). The change to one correct answer in a SATA-style question came at about the same time as scoring them for partial credit instead of all correct or all wrong. These changes came with the launch of the Next Generation Exam in April 2023 (NCSBN, 2024). Employ added techniques for teasing out the answer by underlining important points to the question or highlighting the key points (Nugent & Vitale, 2021-2022).

Use the following strategies for SATA multiple choice questions:

- Approach each possible answer as a true/false.
- Only choose the all true or all false options depending on the wording of the question.
- Stay focused on the question and what it asks.
- Employ multiple testing techniques.

### Matrix Multiple Choice

This is a style of question that has a matrix (a table) with horizontal rows and vertical columns. The tester chooses one option from each row or column. The Electronic Health Record (EHR) can be used to look up data that may help the tester with each portion of the question. Strategies include those that help with straight multiple-choice questions:

- Approach each line as a separate question.
- Cover the portions not needed to decrease distraction and anxiety about the multifaceted style.

### Multiple Response – Select *N*:

This style question tells the tester how many selections to make, such as, "Select 3 medications that the nurse anticipates may be ordered." This requires the tester to consider the side effects, indications, and diagnoses for the medications. The tester can toggle through the information in the EHR to aid in answering the question. Other strategies include

- Narrow down what each choice contributes to the solution.
- Cover the choices that you eliminate
- Ensure your selected answers match the required number of answers in the question (i.e., do not choose 3 answers if the stem requests 4).

**Drop Down Cloze**

A Cloze question is a fill-in-the-blank style question that uses a drop down to finish the statement or answer the question(s) that come with a paragraph of information. Treating these like individual multiple-choice questions will help you choose the correct answer. The question can include multiple sentences that each require an answer, which calls for viewing each sentence individually. This style of question requires you to review each short question and to relate it to the original, overarching question, which can become confusing. Other strategies for this style of question include

- Reading carefully
- Speaking the original question and the sentences in your mind is helpful
- If scrap paper is admissible, request a piece of paper
- Cover the other parts in the grouping and focus on one portion at a time.
- Employ multiple testing techniques.

### True/False with Correction

This is a style of true/false question that requires the tester to identify the portion that is false and make the correction. These can present in a variety of ways, such as word-only questions, photos with questions, and charts with associated questions. Reading and rereading is important before jumping into the answer; be sure to survey the whole item. Having the option to correct alone can pose the possibility that it is false in the tester's mind via the power of suggestion. This style ensures testers' knowledge by requiring them to correct the statement (Nugent & Vitale, 2012-2022).

### Drag and Drop Cloze

This is a fill-in-the-blank style question in which the answers to the incomplete statement are provided and can be dragged into the box to complete the statement. This style gives the tester potential answers versus using data recall to fill in the blank test items. However, style prevents the tester from guessing the answer based on a word's part of speech. This encourages the test writer to mix up the distractors to emphasize critical thinking.

### Drop Down Table

This is a table that has columns that drop down for choices, though a major difference to other types of drop downs is that each column can have more than one answer. This can be as simple as choosing a drug class and patient teaching for a list of medications. Key tip is to take your time.

**Drop Down Rationale**

This style question is based on cause and effect. An EHR with information and a statement with one cause and 1-2 effects that the drop down allows the tester to choose from in order to come to the answer. The biggest key is to read it all first, then decide what the statement is seeking and what clues there are within the EHR.

Treat these like basic multiple-choice questions once the EHR is reviewed

**Bow Tie**

Bow Tie questions include center, right, and left sections. The center is a health concern, the left contains suggested actions, and the right contains parameters to monitor. "Bow-tie questions are among the most challenging of the new NGN question types because they measure all six steps of the clinical judgment measurement model in one question. But not all candidates will see a bow-tie question on the updated exam. Only candidates who continue to test after the minimum-length exam (85 questions) will receive a scored bow-tie question" (UWorld Nursing, para 2, 2023).

- Calm down.
- Read the item carefully.
- Determine the goal/need based on the center item.
- Break the columns into sections and move through each part to finish answering the item.
- Employ multiple testing techniques.

### Highlight Text

These questions are based on a case-study format. Information is given and the tester highlights the requested portions. If an action is needed, the tester must select an intervention. A client could present with a complication and the tester will identify a symptom. The key to the approach for this style is to read carefully and decide what the nurse's intent would be. Understanding the question is crucial; read carefully.

### Highlight Table

These are in a list requiring the tester to highlight the portions that are requested. For instance, a nurse may need to review labs for a patient on Coumadin. The table will contain elements of information from which the tester needs to decide what is relevant or not, requires action or not, and so on. Read carefully and take your time.

### Matching

Matching questions present two columns of information and require the tester to match the items according to the directions. This style can work in your favor if you have the most of the answers in your mind, and then use the process of elimination. Of course, this can backfire if you chose an incorrect response for an item.

- Read directions carefully to ensure you understand the intent of the matching.
- Cover the answer column to determine the answer in your mind.
- Match the items that you know are correct, revealing a

shorter list of options you are not clear on.

- Hopefully, the shorter list reveals more correct responses.
- Resort to an educated guess if the answer is not certain.

**Hot Spot**

Hot Spot questions require the tester to identify a location for an item in a graph, table, or picture. Generally, these questions include anatomy or physiology information to allow the tester to demonstrate that they know how to locate particular aspects pertaining to the model or graph.

- Identify what the question is asking.
- Test the marker to see if it is on the desired portion of the picture or graph.
- Identify landmarks as needed.

In general, practice is the best way to improve and answer the varied types of questions available on the NCLEX. "Practice exams aren't just good for introducing you to more content and giving you a better idea of what you should be studying. They'll also familiarize you with the NCLEX itself, which can make the actual exam much less daunting. So, in the months leading up to your exam date, find a quiet place several times a week and take as many practice tests as you can. The more questions that you can review, the more prepared you will be for the real thing" (Joyce University of Nursing & Health Sciences, p. 29, 2022).

The more familiar a tester can be with the material, the less likely they will feel surprised because the format will be constant and only the topic will change. Programs such as Kaplan or ATI Testing LLC can offer NCLEX style exams that predict the likelihood of passing. While these tools are expensive for individuals, programs like UWorld have affordable options that provide the questions, and the format of the screen within the application is identical to the screen for NCLEX, further aiding in comfort with the exam as just another day of practice questions, according to students who invested in the UWorld program.

- **What platforms will your school offer for practice questions?**
- **How are you at prioritizing your study time?**
- **Do you need to set a schedule that includes practice question time?**

# Chapter 7: I Would NEVER Cheat!

Do not cheat or plagiarize! It's difficult to think it might be an issue in this field, but it is real. The reason for doing it does not matter; cheating or plagiarizing is a major red flag indicating that you will be a person who would compromise good nursing practice at the risk of the patient.

Before getting offended at the possible suggestion of such a thing, understand that cheating and the resulting health-care compromise is a national phenomenon across the country. A general evolution of thought is that students cheat more with the access to electronic resources because students do not consider copying from the internet cheating (Emmanuel et al., 2021). This is especially problematic in the study of nursing because almost all nursing documentation and research is electronic. While cheating in nursing dates as far back as the 1900's, the prevalence seems to be tied to perception of the definition of cheating.

Students who cheat in the classroom are more likely to cheat in the clinical setting regardless of the impact or risk to the patient according to Žvanut (2022). Even more problematic is, "In cases where students deliberately fail to demonstrate academic integrity during their student years, evidence indicates a higher likelihood that they will also act dishonestly in the workplace (Emmanuel et al, p. 51, 2021).

Students attribute their reasoning for poor decisions around cheating to stress, family difficulty, time constraints, lack of knowledge, and feeling overwhelmed. Most commonly, excuses for cheating include statements like, "I have never done anything like this before. I would never do something like this in clinical or when I am a nurse." However, the cited articles assert that this rationale is far from the truth; it is more likely that cheating occurred previously and is more likely to occur in the future based on the lack of integrity and critical thinking involved in the act at hand (Žvanut, 2022).

To avoid cheating, do not consider short cuts. Laziness, which cheating usually boils down to, is dangerous to you as a student, as an employee, and to your patients. Thinking you will get away with it "this time" is a dangerous strategy. Imagine telling your family and friends why you no longer attend nursing school or why you got fired from your job or what that lawsuit is about. Worse yet, imagine harming a patient because you cut corners. Cheating on the NCLEX nursing board exam is not possible, so cheating during your nursing education reduces your chance of success on those boards.

There is some shared responsibility however on the part of the faculty and nursing program. According to Emmanuel et al., (2021), a program has the responsibility of embedding academic honesty and integrity within the courses beginning with the very first semester. Providing opportunities for practicing ethical decision making is considered a baseline for programs given the widespread increase in documented cheating nationwide.

- **How do you think programs can best prepare students with this?**
- **What is your personal definition of cheating or plagiarism?**
- **What would your response be to a classmate cheating?**

# Conclusion

The first step to nursing school should not be the NCLEX; that is the final step. Nursing school will contain coursework and evaluations (tests) in ascending difficulty that will prepare the student for, not just that "final step," but for a satisfying and successful career. A good nursing program will follow a curriculum that will mold and shape each student into a knowledgeable, professional, ethical, collaborative, and patient-focused novice practitioner.

Nursing education, in addition to regular classwork and evaluation, should include a variety of opportunities to work with fellow students and the target population of injured and ill patients. Learning activities will include papers, class assignments, group work, and tests; clinical and community support opportunities.

The program should construct exams to offer varied examples of question styles to increase students' ability to perform well on these items in preparation for the "final step." Additionally, understanding the test format structure, such as ADPIE or Bloom's Taxonomy, helps direct the tester to item development to understand the "what" of the question. When the tester can narrow down the intent of the question, regardless of the format, and make answering it more straightforward. Practicing the steps in Chapter 5 cannot guarantee a passing result. The tester requires a positive mindset, and methods for performing well under stress. Jelinik & Richards (2022) note that employing positive self-talk is beneficial on many levels, saying, "people who engage in positive self-talk developed effective strategies to cope with their emotions and mental stress" (para 8). Positive self-talk is an internal dialogue that makes a person feel good about themselves. A person can use positive self-talk to think optimistically and feel motivated. Identifying negative self-talk is the first step toward thinking more positively" (Jelinik & Richards, para 1, 2022).

Consider finding a tutor. Over the course of nearly 20 years of educating nursing students, I observed that the most successful students proactively sought a tutor. They reported that a tutor helped them organize their thoughts so they could think through and verbalize the concepts.

Addressing mindset, exercise, positive study habits, organization, and the professional writing skills help the learner to expand their approach to learning by identifying gaps in facts and knowledge. Finally, working through practice tests and using multiple strategies to answer questions is mentioned as an effective strategy by several of the authors within the reference list. In general, practicing is the key to success. Practice holding a positive mindset, practice professionalism, practice different approaches to studying, and practice actively engaging with your learning in a variety of ways.

Thank you for reading this book. After you complete nursing school, email me and tell me which part of this book was the most helpful. phillips5mary@gmail.com.

# References

[illegible]

# References

Ahmad, M., Aboud, A., and Manna, B. (2023). Wound Pressure Injury Management. StatPearls Publishing; 2024 Jan. https://pubmed.ncbi.nlm.nih.gov/30422492/

Barrie, L. (2024). Everyday Health. https://www.everydayhealth.com/diet-nutrition-pictures/the-healthiest-power-fruits-next-door.aspx

Bauer, D., Kopp, V., Fischer, M. R. (2007). Answer changing in multiple choice assessment change that answer when in doubt--and spread the word! National Library of Medicine. Pub Med. https://pubmed.ncbi.nlm.nih.gov/17718902/Chamberlain University, May 22, 2023. https://www.chamberlain.edu/blog/6-tips-for-a-successful-nursing-school-study-group

Berg, Eric MD, 2014. How to LOWER cortisol levels? Retrieved March 19, 2024 from https://www.youtube.com/watch?v=L2fKo_dbXS0 Concordia University Texas, 2022. Self Care for nursing students: 9 tips. Retrieved on May 9, 2024 from https://absn.concordia.edu/blog/self-care-for-nursing-students/#:~:text=Self%2Dcare%20practices%20among%20nursing,and%20interacting%20with%20loved%20ones.

Emmanuel, Elizabeth, Fielden, Jann, Miller-Rosser, Kolleen, 2021. Why should we care about academic integrity in nursing students? Journal of Nursing Education and Practice. Retrieved 2/13/24 file:///Users/maryphillips/Downloads/19714-67424-1-PB.pdf

Gepp, Karin and Lovering, Cathy, March 31, 2022. How personality can affect stress levels. Psych Central. Retrieved March 14, 2024 from: https://psychcentral.com/lib/stress-and-personality

Haury, Corissa, November 23, 2022. Why writing by hand is still the best way to retain information. https://stackoverflow.blog/2022/11/23/why-writing-by-hand-is-still-the-best-way-to-retain-information/.

Joyce University of Nursing & Health Sciences, 04/11/2022. 49 Proven NCLEX Strategies. Retrieved 03/11/2024 from: https://www.joyce.edu/wp-content/uploads/2022/04/49-Proven-NCLEX-Strategies-eBook.pdf

Manjit Kaur Khaira, Raja Lexshimi Raja Gopal, Suriati Mohamed Saini, and Zaleha Md Isa, 2023. Interventional Strategies to Reduce Test Anxiety among Nursing Students: A Systematic Review.

Jelinik, J. & Richards, L. March 18, 2022. Medical News Today. What is Positive Self Talk? Retrieved 3/13/24 from: https://www.medicalnewstoday.com/articles/positive-self-talk

Kristi Depaul, February 2, 2021 https://hbr.org/2021/02/what-does-it-really-take-to-build-a-new-habit

Loveless, Becton, 2024. Test Taking Strategies for Nursing Students. Education Corner. Retrieved 2/15/24 https://www.educationcorner.com/nursing-test-taking-strategies/#:~:text=Answer%20the%20question%20in%20your,answer%20is%20the%20correct%20answer.

NCSBN, 2024. Retrieved 2/28/24 from, National Council of State Boards of Nursing Inc., https://ncsbn.zendesk.com/hc/en-us/articles/7807140341143-What-types-of-items-were-approved-for-the-Next-Generation-NCLEX

NCSBN, 2023. Retrieved 3/5/24 from The Next Generation NCLEX, NCLEX-RN Test Plan. https://www.ncsbn.org/public-files/2023_RN_Test%20Plan_English_FINAL.pdf Purdue University, 2024. General Format. https://owl.purdue.edu/owl/research_and_citation/apa_style/apa_style_introduction.html

Purdue University Global, 2024. The Importance of Self-Care for Nurses and How to Put a Plan in Place. Retrieved on 4/23/24 from: https://www.purdueglobal.edu/blog/nursing/self-care-for-nurses/

Richmond, Jennifer, 2024. https://nursester.com/is-recording-nursing-school-lectures-a-good-or-bad-idea/

Ross, Paul, 2019. Novice To Expert: Constructivism in Nursing Adult Learning, Nurse Educator. Retrieved on 2/14/24 https://nursingeducationnetwork.net/2019/04/24/novice-to-expert-constructivism-in-nursing/

Shah, Matali, para 9, 2022. https://www.harpersbazaar.in/culture/story/heres-why-watching-the-same-tv-show-and-movie-over-and-over-again-is-so-comforting-564387-2022-08-08

Speedyprep, 2023, May, 26, 2020 https://speedyprep.com/7-benefits-of-study-groups/

UWorld, May 14, 2121 https://nursing.uworld.com/blog/growth-mindset-can-lead-to-nursing-school-success/

UWorld Nursing, April 12, 2023. https://nursing.uworld.com/blog/tips-for-answering-bow-tie-questions/

Whitworth, Nicole, 2024. How (and Why!) to find nursing school help. Retrieved 3/20/24 from https://www.yournursingtutor.com/how-to-find-nursing-school-help/

Žvanut, B., 2022. Profiling nursing students' dishonest behaviour: Classroom versus clinical settings. Retrieved 2/13/24 https://www.ncbi.nlm.nih.gov/pmc/articles/PMC9527370/